DIABETIC COOKBOOK FOR BEGINNER

Easy and Healthy low-sugar Recipes

Gena **miller**

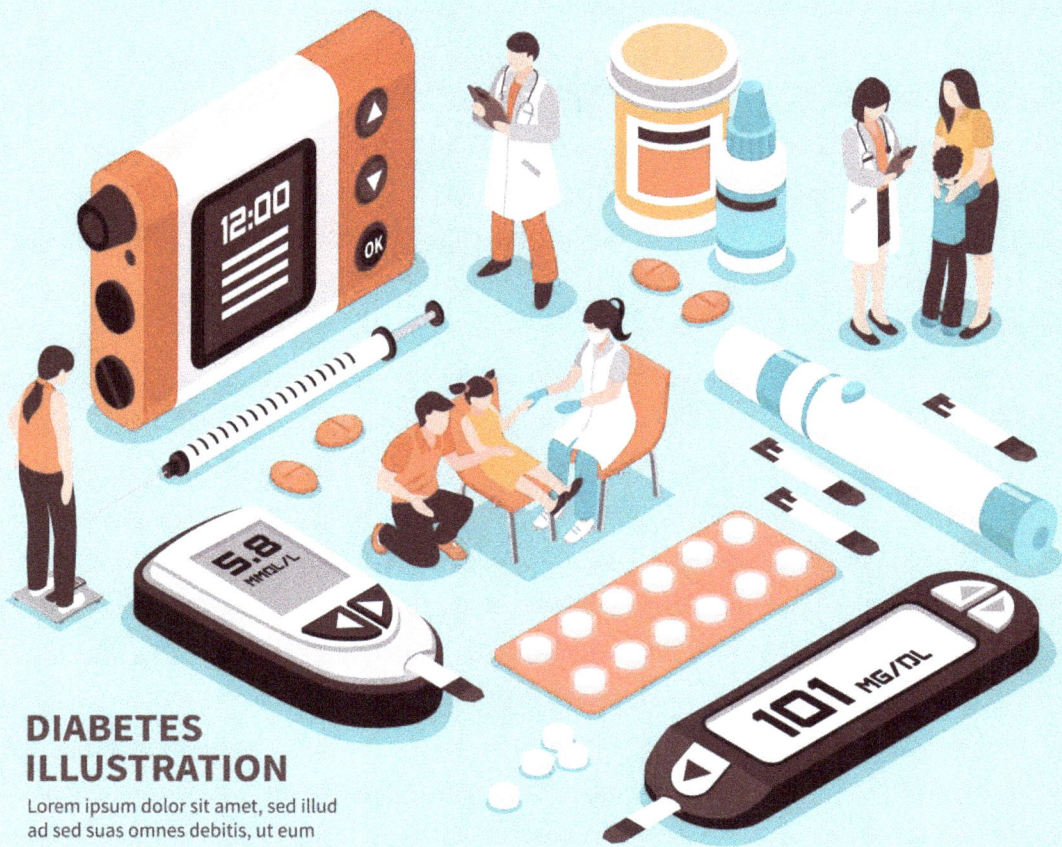

DIABETES ILLUSTRATION

Lorem ipsum dolor sit amet, sed illud
ad sed suas omnes debitis, ut eum

Table Of Content:

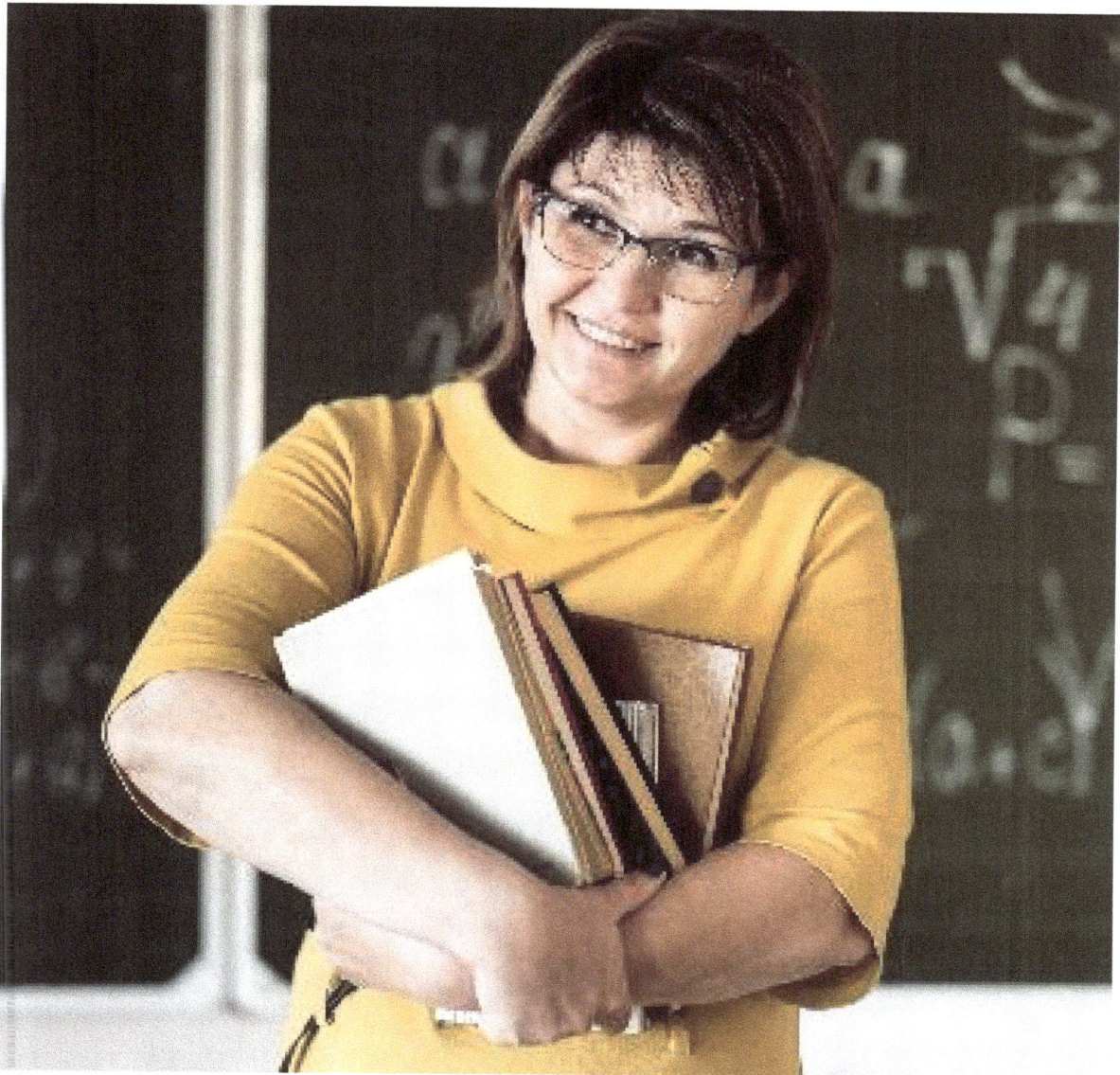

Gena Miller was born in Portland Oregon in 1970 to a wealthy family, Gena has the opportunity to continue her studies away from home, thanks to the economic aid of her father, and for this reason, she decided to attend the renowned university "Columbia University in New York". She had no difficulty in graduating in 1998 with top marks, winning a scholarship in "nutritional sciences" which allowed her to find a job at the university as a lecturer. Gena took her profession very much to heart and saw in teaching the possibility of giving her students the necessary tools to establish a healthy and wholesome lifestyle, drawing up for them real nutritional plans with tasty and healthy recipes. It was her students who encouraged her to start writing "health and wellness" books. The first books were a success and were a stimulus for many people so Gena soon became a successful writer, her experience and love for others led her to understand the real needs of people with food problems and the difficulties they had in approaching food, Gena managed more and more to give the right amount of nutritional value and good taste to her dishes creating delicious and easy recipes appreciated by all.

Introdution

Diabetes is a disease that affects many people, both young and old. So, how can you live a healthy life with this condition? What is the impact on your diet, exercise regimen and daily life? Eating healthy is an important part of diabetes management because it lowers blood sugar levels. This diabetic beginner's cookbook has all the recipes, from appetizers to desserts, to help you eat the right way. Managing diabetes takes a lot of planning, and a great diet is the key to a healthy lifestyle. Following a nutritious diet means eating the right foods and avoiding empty calories. A healthy, balanced diet will help you lose weight and avoid complications like heart disease. But here are some things you shouldn't eat if you have diabetes: Sugary foods like cakes, pastries and sugary snacks like sweets should be avoided. You need to replace them with healthier choices like fruit or cereal bars. Skipping meals can significantly increase blood sugar levels. For this reason, it is important to eat regular meals. Fast food is a no-no because it is usually high in saturated fat and carbohydrates. A healthier alternative would be grilled fish or chicken and vegetables cooked in olive or sunflower oil and served with a yogurt sauce. High-fat dairy products should be avoided because they can drastically increase blood sugar levels. Instead, choose low-fat dairy products like cheese and yogurt or eat more beans and nuts. Sugary drinks such as soda and fruit juice should be avoided if possible. Opt for water instead. If you're craving a drink, opt for something like orange juice diluted with a slice of lime, which is much healthier. When cooking for yourself, use olive oil instead of sunflower or vegetable oil. Always make sure and keep your body hydrated by drinking plenty of water. Don't drink too much, as you would with a hangover. A general rule of thumb is to drink at least 2/3 of your body weight in ounces, but you should check with your doctor before doing this. Water is a very important part of a healthy lifestyle and it's easy to get carried away in the heat. It helps you cool down. If you can't go to the supermarket for groceries every day, then try to buy some staples like fish or canned vegetables for convenience. If you're worried about the cost of eating healthy, visit your local supermarket's website to plan your weekly grocery shopping. Compare prices and items among chains or supermarkets in your area. Planning will also help you avoid getting carried away with impulse purchases. If you have diabetes, planning a healthy diet is essential for several reasons: It helps prevent complications such as heart disease and stroke. It helps you lose weight. It makes sure you get vitamins and minerals from the food you eat. Controlling your blood sugar levels is also very important when managing diabetes. Your body needs insulin to control the amount of sugar in your blood, as it is essential for your cells to use or store glucose for energy. The correct level of insulin is a key factor in controlling blood sugar levels and stabilizing them. A healthy diet is made up of many foods with carbohydrates to provide energy. Carbohydrates are found in fruits and vegetables, as well as whole grain bread, pasta and rice. High-carbohydrate foods are usually not rich in nutrients. They can also be used as a quick source of useful energy for the brain, especially during exercise or when feeling tired. These carbohydrates are mainly found in things like bread, sugar and junk food like cakes, cookies and pies. They should be avoided because they are usually high in saturated fat and sugar, and can raise blood sugar levels dramatically. Protein is essential for growth. They are found in meat, chicken, fish, eggs and dairy products. Protein makes you feel full longer. To get the most out of your diet, combine a carbohydrate meal with a small amount of protein such as lean meat or fish to balance blood sugar levels and keep you feeling full until the next meal. Saturated fats can increase bad cholesterol levels, so try to avoid saturated fats like butter and palm oil. You should replace them with unsaturated fats like olive oil. Unsalted nuts contain a lot of fat and can replace fatty snacks and foods, helping you watch what you eat and giving you the nutrients your body needs.

Breakfast

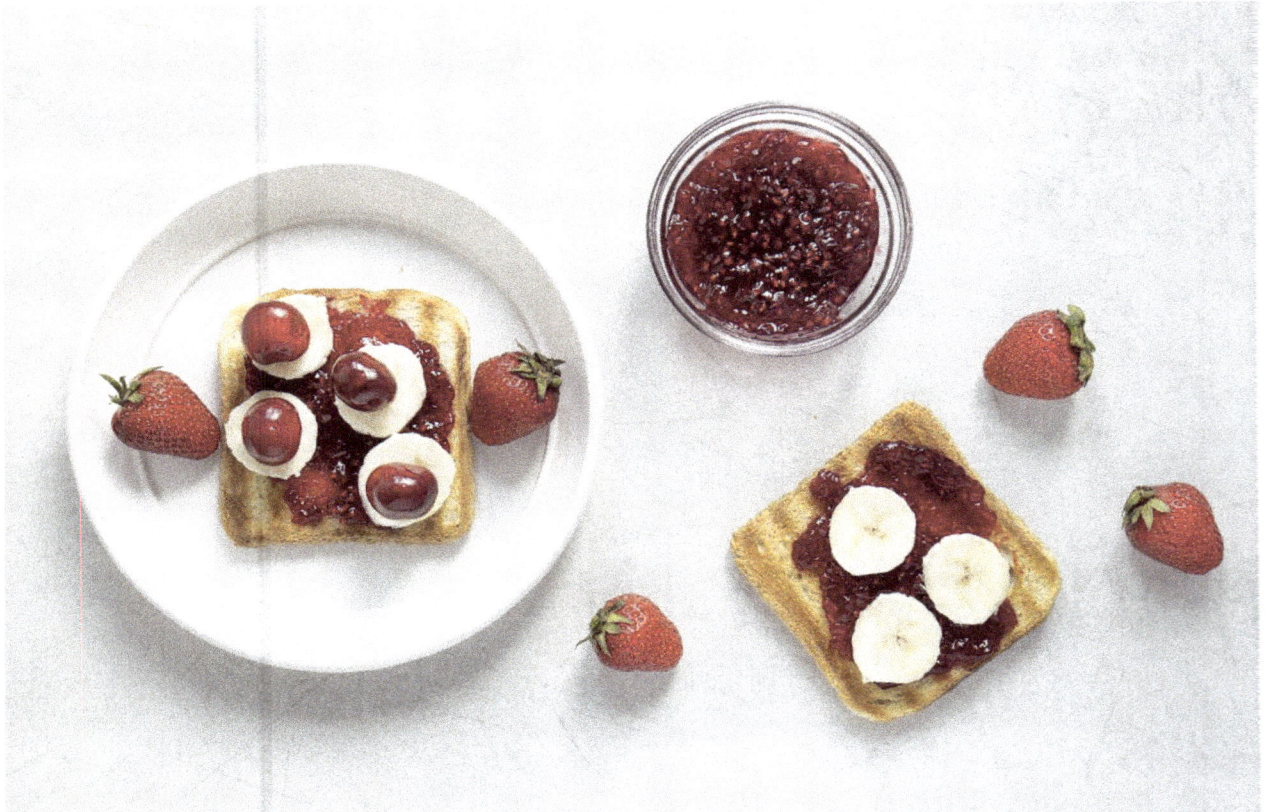

Yogurt Sundae

Prep time: 5 minutes

Cook time: 0 minutes

Serves 1

Ingredients:

- ¾ cup plain nonfat Greek yogurt
- ¼ cup mixed berries (blueberries, strawberries, blackberries)
- 2 tablespoons cashew, walnut, or almond pieces
- 1 tablespoon ground flaxseed
- 2 fresh mint leaves,

Instruction:

1. shredded Spoon the yogurt into a small bowl.
2. Top with the berries, nuts, and flaxseed.
3. Garnish with the mint and serve.

Nutrition fats : calories: 238 | fat: 11g | protein: 21g | carbs: 16g | sugars: 9g | fiber: 4g | sodium: 64mg

Breakfast Egg Bites

Prep time: 10 minutes

Cook time: 25 minutes

Serves 8

Ingredients:

- Nonstick cooking spray 6 eggs, beaten
- ¼ cup unsweetened plain almond milk
- 1 red bell pepper, diced
- 1 cup chopped spinach
- ¼ cup crumbled goat cheese
- ½ cup sliced brown mushrooms
- ¼ cup sliced sun-dried tomatoes Salt and freshly ground black pepper, to taste

Instructions:

1. Preheat the oven to 350°F (180°C).
2. Spray 8 muffin cups of a 12-cup muffin tin with nonstick cooking spray.
3. Set aside.
4. In a large mixing bowl, combine the eggs, almond milk, bell pepper, spinach, goat cheese, mushrooms, and tomatoes.
5. Season with salt and pepper.
6. Fill the prepared muffin cups three-fourths full with the egg mixture.
7. Bake for 20 to 25 minutes until the eggs are set.
8. Let cool slightly and remove the egg bites from the muffin tin.
9. Serve warm, or store in an airtight container in the refrigerator for up to 5 days or in the freezer for up to 1 month.

Nutrition facts: Per Serving calories: 68 | fat: 4g | protein: 6g | carbs: 3g | sugars: 2g | fiber: 1g | sodium: 126mg

Savory Corn Grits

Prep time: 5 minutes

Cook time: 7 minutes

Serves 4

Ingredients:

- 2 cups water
- 1 cup fat-free milk
- 1 cup stone-ground corn grits

Instructions:

1. In a heavy-bottomed pot, bring the water and milk to a simmer over medium heat.
2. Gradually add the grits, stirring continuously.
3. Reduce the heat to low, cover, and cook, stirring often, for 5 to 7 minutes, or until the grits are soft and tender.
4. Serve and enjoy.

Nutrition facts: Per Serving calories: 166 | fat: 1g | protein: 6g | carbs: 34g | sugars: 3g | fiber: 1g | sodium: 32mg

Blueberry Coconut Breakfast Cookies

Prep time: 10 minutes

Cook time: 15 minutes

Serves 4

Ingredients:

- 4 tablespoons unsalted butter, at room temperature
- 2 medium bananas
- 4 large eggs
- ½ cup unsweetened applesauce
- 1 teaspoon vanilla extract
- ⅔ cup coconut flour ¼ teaspoon salt
- 1 cup fresh or frozen blueberries

Instructions:

1. Preheat the oven to 375°F (190°C).
2. In a medium bowl, mash the butter and bananas together with a fork until combined.
3. The bananas can be a little chunky.
4. Add the eggs, applesauce, and vanilla to the bananas and mix well.
5. Stir in the coconut flour and salt.
6. Gently fold in the blueberries.
7. Drop about 2 tablespoons of dough on a baking sheet for each cookie and flatten it a bit with the back of a spoon.
8. Bake for about 13 minutes, or until firm to the touch.

Nutrition facts: Per Serving calories: 305 | fat: 18g | protein: 8g | carbs: 28g | sugars: 15g | fiber: 7g | sodium: 222mg

Toads in Holes

Prep time: 5 minutes

Cook time: 5 minutes

Serves 2

Ingredients:

- 2 tablespoons butter
- 2 slices whole-wheat bread
- 2 large eggs

Instructions:

1. Sea salt and freshly ground black pepper, to taste In a medium nonstick skillet over medium heat, heat the butter until it bubbles.
2. As the butter heats, cut a 3-inch hole in the middle of each piece of bread. Discard the centers.
3. Place the bread pieces in the butter in the pan.
4. Carefully crack an egg into the hole of each piece of bread.
5. Cook until the bread crisps and the egg whites set, about 3 minutes.
6. Flip and cook just until the yolk is almost set, 1 to 2 minutes more.
7. Season to taste with the salt and pepper.

Nutrition facts: Per Serving calories: 241 | fat: 17g | protein: 10g | carbs: 12g | sugars: cg | fiber: 2g | sodium: 307mg

Walnut and Oat Granola

Prep time: 10 minutes

Cook time: 30 minutes

Serves: 16

Ingredients:

- 4 cups rolled oats
- 1 cup walnut pieces
- ½ cup pepitas
- ¼ teaspoon salt
- 1 teaspoon ground cinnamon
- 1 teaspoon ground ginger
- ½ cup coconut oil, melted
- ½ cup unsweetened applesauce
- 1 teaspoon vanilla extract
- ½ cup dried cherries

Instruction :

1. Preheat the oven to 350°F (180°C).
2. Line a baking sheet with parchment paper.
3. In a large bowl, toss the oats, walnuts, pepitas, salt, cinnamon, and ginger.
4. In a large measuring cup, combine the coconut oil, applesauce, and vanilla.
5. Pour over the dry mixture and mix well.
6. Transfer the mixture to the prepared baking sheet.

7. Cook for 30 minutes, stirring about halfway through.

8. Remove from the oven and let the granola sit undisturbed until completely cool.

9. Break the granola into pieces, and stir in the dried cherries.

10. Transfer to an airtight container, and store at room temperature for up to 2 weeks.

Nutrition facts: per Serving: calories: 225 fat: 14.9g protein: 4.9g carbs: 20.1g fiber: 3.1g sugar: 4.9g sodium: 31mg

Apple and Bran Muffins

Prep time: 10 minutes

Cook time: 20 minutes

Serves: 18 muffins

Ingredients:

- 2 cups whole-wheat flour
- 1 cup wheat bran
- 1/3 cup granulated sweetener
- 1 tablespoon baking powder
- 2 teaspoons ground cinnamon
- ½ teaspoon ground ginger
- ¼ teaspoon ground nutmeg Pinch sea salt
- 2 eggs
- 1½ cups skim milk, at room temperature
- ½ cup melted coconut oil
- 2 teaspoons pure vanilla extract 2
- apples, peeled, cored, and diced

Instructions:

1. Preheat the oven to 350°F (180°C).
2. Line 18 muffin cups with paper liners and set the tray aside.
3. In a large bowl, stir together the flour, bran, sweetener, baking powder, cinnamon, ginger, nutmeg, and salt.
4. In a small bowl, whisk the eggs, milk, coconut oil, and vanilla until blended.
5. Add the wet ingredients to the dry ingredients, stirring until just blended.

6. Stir in the apples and spoon equal amounts of batter into each muffin cup.
7. Bake the muffins until a toothpick inserted in the center of a muffin comes out clean, about 20 minutes.
8. Cool the muffins completely and serve.
9. Store leftover muffins in a sealed container in the refrigerator for up to 3 days or in the freezer for up to 1 month.

Nutrition facts: per Serving: calories: 142 fat: 7.1g protein: 4.1g carbs: 19.1g fiber: 3.1g sugar: 6.1g sodium: 21mg

Greek Yogurt and Oat Pancakes

Prep time: 5 minutes

Cook time: 20 minutes

Serves: 4

Ingredients:

- 1 cup 2 percent plain Greek yogurt
- 3 eggs
- 1½ teaspoons pure vanilla extract
- 1 cup rolled oats
- 1 tablespoon granulated sweetener
- 1 teaspoon baking powder
- 1 teaspoon ground cinnamon Pinch ground cloves
- Nonstick cooking spray

Instruction:

1. Place the yogurt, eggs, and vanilla in a blender and pulse to combine.
2. Add the oats, sweetener, baking powder, cinnamon, and cloves to the blender and blend until the batter is smooth.
3. Place a large nonstick skillet over medium heat and lightly coat it with cooking spray.
4. Spoon ¼ cup of batter per pancake, 4 at a time, into the skillet.
5. Cook the pancakes until the bottoms are firm and golden, about 4 minutes.
6. Flip the pancakes over and cook the other side until they are cooked through, about 3 minutes.
7. Remove the pancakes to a plate and repeat with the remaining batter.

8. Serve with fresh fruit.

Nutrition facts: per Serving: calories: 244 fat: 8.1g protein: 13.1g carbs: 28.1g fiber: 4.0g sugar: 3.0g sodium: 82mg

Asparagus Frittata

Prep time: 12 minutes

Cook time: 45 minutes

Serves: 6

Ingredients:

- 1 lb. of thin asparagus
- 2 onions, chopped
- 1 ½ teaspoons extra-virgin olive oil
- 1 red bell pepper, chopped
- 2 cloves garlic, minced
- ½ cup of water
- 4 large eggs
- 2 large egg whites
- 1 cup part-skim ricotta cheese
- ½ teaspoon sea salt, divided
- 1 tablespoon parsley, fresh chopped
- ½ cup Gruyere cheese, shredded
- 2 tablespoons breadcrumbs, dry

Instructions:

1. Preheat your oven to 325° Fahrenheit.
2. Coat a 10-inch pie pan with some cooking spray.
3. Sprinkle pan with breadcrumbs.
4. Remove the tough ends of the asparagus: slice tips off and reserve.

5. Slice the asparagus stalks into 1/2-inch-long slices.

6. Heat your oil in a nonstick pan over medium-high heat.

7. Next, add the bell pepper, onions, garlic and ¼ teaspoon sea salt.

8. Cook for 7 minutes.

9. Add water to the asparagus stalks in the pan and cook while stirring until asparagus is tender, for about 7 minutes or until the liquid is evaporated.

10. Season with salt and pepper as needed, arranging the vegetables in an even layer in the pan.

11. Whisk your egg whites and eggs in a mixing bowl.

12. Add the ricotta, parsley and remaining sea salt and pepper, then whisk to blend.

13. Pour your egg mixture over the vegetables in the pan while gently shaking the pan to distribute evenly.

14. Scatter your reserved asparagus tips over the top along with the Gruyere.

15. Bake your frittata until a knife inserted in the middle comes out clean.

16. It should take about 35 minutes.

17. Let your frittata stand for about 5 minutes before serving.

18. Serve and enjoy!

Nutrition facts: (per 1/6 of recipe): Calories: 193 Fat: 11g Protein: 15g Carbs: 10g

Whole-Grain Dutch Baby Pancake

Prep Time: 5 minutes

Cook Time: 25 minutes

Serves: 4

Ingredients:

- 2 tablespoons coconut oil
- 1/2 cup whole-wheat flour
- ¼ cup skim milk
- 3 large eggs
- 1 teaspoon vanilla extract
- 1/2 teaspoon baking powder
- ¼ teaspoon salt
- ¼ teaspoon ground cinnamon
- Powdered sugar, for dusting

Instructions:

1. Preheat the oven to 400f.
2. Put the coconut oil in a medium oven-safe skillet, and place the skillet in the oven to melt the oil while it preheats.
3. In a blender, combine the flour, milk, eggs, vanilla, baking powder, salt, and cinnamon.
4. Process until smooth.
5. Carefully remove the skillet from the oven and tilt to spread the oil around evenly.

6. Pour the batter into the skillet and return it to the oven for 23 to 25 minutes, until the pancake puffs and lightly browns.
7. Remove, dust lightly with powdered sugar, cut into 4 wedges, and serve.

Nutrition Facts: Calories: 195; Total Fat: 11g; Saturated Fat: 7g; Protein: 8g; Carbs: 16g; Sugar: 1g; Fiber: 2g; Cholesterol: 140mg; Sodium: 209mg

Lovely Porridge

Prep Time: 15 minutes

Cook Time: Nil

Serves: 2

Ingredients:

- 2 tablespoons coconut flour
- 2 tablespoons vanilla protein powder
- 3 tablespoons Golden Flaxseed meal
- 1 and 1/2 cups almond milk, unsweetened
- Powdered erythritol

Instructions:

1. Take a bowl and mix in flaxseed meal, protein powder, coconut flour and mix well
2. Add mix to the saucepan (placed over medium heat)
3. Add almond milk and stir, let the mixture thicken
4. Add your desired amount of sweetener and serve
5. Enjoy!

Nutrition facts: Calories: 259; Fat: 13g; Carbohydrates: 5g; Protein: 16g

Greek Chicken Breast

Prep Time: 10 minutes

Cook Time: 25 minutes

Serves: 4

Ingredients:

- 4 chicken breast halves, skinless and boneless
- 1 cup extra virgin olive oil
- 1 lemon, juiced
- 2 teaspoons garlic, crushed
- 1 and 1/2 teaspoons black pepper
- 1/3 teaspoon paprika

Instructions:

1. Cut 3 slits in the chicken breast
2. Take a small bowl and whisk in olive oil, salt, lemon juice, garlic, paprika, pepper and whisk for 30 seconds
3. Place chicken in a large bowl and pour marinade
4. Rub the marinade all over using your hand Refrigerate overnight
5. Pre-heat grill to medium heat and oil the grate
6. Cook chicken in the grill until center is no longer pink
7. Serve and enjoy!

Nutrition facts: Calories: 644; Fat: 57g; Carbohydrates: 2g; Protein: 27g

Breakfast Salad

Prep Time: 5 minutes

Cook Time: 15 minutes

Serves: 3

Ingredients:

- 1 cup finely diced kale
- 1 cup cabbage, red and Chinese
- 2 tbsp. coconut oil
- 1 cup spinach
- 2 moderate avocados
- 1.2kg chickpeas sprout
- 2 tbsp. sunflower seed sprouts
- Pure sea salt (seasoning)
- Bell pepper (seasoning)
- Lemon juice (seasoning)

Instructions:

1. Add spinach, Chinese and red cabbage, kale, coconut oil, to a container.
2. Add seasoning to taste and mix adequately.
3. Add other ingredients and mix.

Nutrition facts: Calories: 112 Protein: 28g Fiber: 10g Sugar: 1g

Cheese Yogurt

Prep Time: 12 minutes

Cook Time: 15 minutes

Serves: 2

Ingredients:

- 1 thick and Creamy Yogurt or store-bought yogurt
- ½ tsp. kosher salt

Instructions:

1. Line a strainer of twice the normal or plastic cheesecloth thickness.
2. Place the strainer on top of a bowl and apply the yogurt.
3. Cover and refrigerate for 2 hours.
4. Stir in the salt and continue to drip for another 2 hours until the yogurt cheese is ready to spread.

Nutrition facts: Calories: 83 Protein: 5g Fat: 5.4g

Breakfast Cake

Prep time: 5 minutes

Cook time: 45 minutes

Serves: 4

Ingredients:

- Coconut flour, 1/2 cup
- Vanilla protein powder, 3-4 tablespoons
- Baking soda, 1/2 teaspoon
- Salt, 1/8 teaspoon
- Eggs, 6
- Olive oil, 1/4 cup
- Water, 3/4 cup
- Baking paper

Instructions:

1. Preheat your oven to 350°Fahrenheit/180°Celsius.
2. Inside a food processor, mix the first 4 items for 10 seconds.
3. Toss in the remaining ingredients until well mixed.
4. Line the lower end and edges of a squared baking tray (20cm/ 8") using baking paper, now pour the flour mixture within the frying pan.
5. Cook for around 60-50 minutes, then remove from oven, allow to cool before serving.

Nutritional Facts: Fat: 12g, Net Carbs: 6g3 Protein: 15g, Sodium: 18mg

Lunch

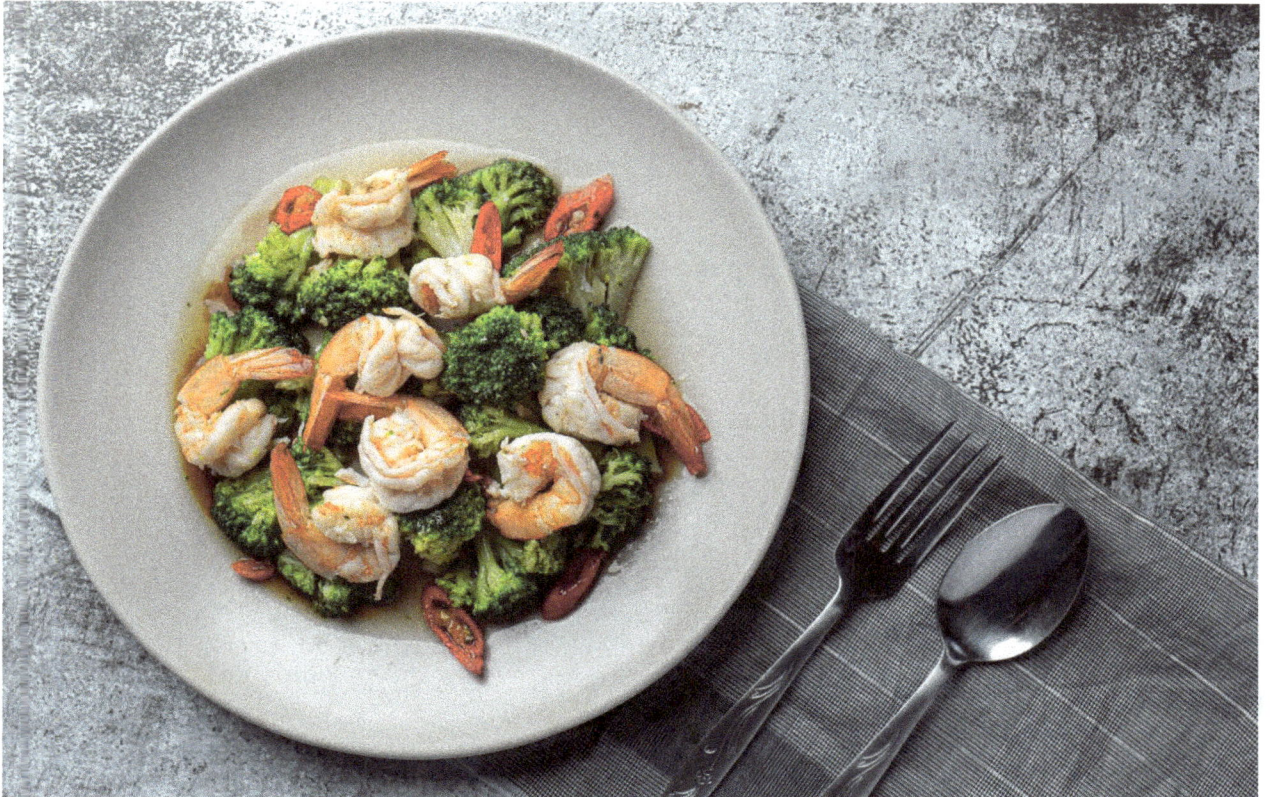

Blueberry and Chicken Salad

Prep Time: 10 minutes

Cook Time: 0 minute

Serves: 4

Ingredients:

- 2 cups chopped cooked chicken
- 1 cup fresh blueberries
- ¼ cup almonds
- 1 celery stalk
- ¼ cup red onion
- 1 tablespoon fresh basil
- 1 tablespoon fresh cilantro
- ½ cup plain, vegan mayonnaise
- ¼ teaspoon salt
- ¼ teaspoon freshly ground black pepper
- 8 cups salad greens

Instructions:

1. Toss chicken, blueberries, almonds, celery, onion, basil, and cilantro.
2. Blend yogurt, salt, and pepper.
3. Stir chicken salad to combine.
4. Situate 2 cups of salad greens on each of 4 plates and divide the chicken salad among the plates to serve.

Nutrition facts: 207 Calories; 11g Carbohydrates; 6g Sugars

Buffalo Chicken Salads

Prep Time: 7 minutes

Cook Time: 3 hours

Serves: 5

Ingredients:

- 1½ pounds chicken breast halves
- ½ cup Wing Time® Buffalo chicken sauce
- 4 teaspoons cider vinegar
- 1 teaspoon Worcestershire sauce
- 1 teaspoon paprika
- 1/3 cup light mayonnaise
- 2 tablespoons fat-free milk
- 2 tablespoons crumbled blue cheese
- 2 romaine hearts, chopped
- 1 cup whole grain croutons
- ½ cup very thinly sliced red onion

Instructions:

1. Place chicken in a 2-quarts slow cooker.
2. Mix together Worcestershire sauce, 2 teaspoons of vinegar and Buffalo sauce in a small bowl; pour over chicken.
3. Dust with paprika.
4. Close and cook for 3 hours on low-heat setting.
5. Mix the leftover 2 teaspoons of vinegar with milk and light mayonnaise together in a small bowl at serving time; mix in blue cheese.
6. While chicken is still in the slow cooker, pull meat into bite-sized pieces using two forks.
7. Split the romaine among 6 dishes.
8. Spoon sauce and chicken over lettuce.
9. Pour with blue cheese dressing then add red onion slices and croutons on top.

Nutrition facts: 274 Calories; 11g Carbohydrate; 2g Fiber

Chicken and Cornmeal Dumplings

Prep Time: 8 minutes

Cook Time: 8 hours

Serves: 4

Ingredients:

- Chicken and Vegetable Filling
- 2 medium carrots, thinly sliced
- 1 stalk celery, thinly sliced
- 1/3 cup corn kernels
- ½ of a medium onion, thinly sliced
- 2 cloves garlic, minced
- 1 teaspoon snipped fresh rosemary
- ¼ teaspoon ground black pepper
- 2 chicken thighs, skinned
- 1 cup reduced sodium chicken broth
- ½ cup fat-free milk
- 1 tablespoon all-purpose flour   Cornmeal Dumplings
- ¼ cup flour
- ¼ cup cornmeal
- ½ teaspoon baking powder
- 1 egg white
- 1 tablespoon fat-free milk

- 1 tablespoon canola oil

Instructions:

1. Mix 1/4 teaspoon pepper, carrots, garlic, celery, rosemary, corn, and onion in a 1 1/2 or 2-quart slow cooker.
2. Place chicken on top.
3. Pour the broth atop mixture in the cooker.
4. Close and cook on low-heat for 7 to 8 hours.
5. If cooking with the low-heat setting, switch to high-heat setting (or if heat setting is not available, continue to cook).
6. Place the chicken onto a cutting board and let to cool slightly.
7. Once cool enough to handle, chop off chicken from bones and get rid of the bones.
8. Chop the chicken and place back into the mixture in cooker.
9. Mix flour and milk in a small bowl until smooth.
10. Stir into the mixture in cooker.
11. Drop the Cornmeal Dumplings dough into 4 mounds atop hot chicken mixture using two spoons.
12. Cover and cook for 20 to 25 minutes more or until a toothpick come out clean when inserted into a dumpling. (Avoid lifting lid when cooking.)
13. Sprinkle each of the serving with coarse pepper if desired.
14. Mix together 1/2 teaspoon baking powder, 1/4 cup flour, a dash of salt and 1/4 cup cornmeal in a medium bowl.
15. Mix 1 tablespoon canola oil, 1 egg white and 1 tablespoon fat-free milk in a small bowl.
16. Pour the egg mixture into the flour mixture.
17. Mix just until moistened.

Nutrition facts: 369 Calories; 9g Sugar; 47g Carbohydrate

Moroccan Eggplant Stew

Prep time: 20 minutes

Cook time: 3 minutes

Serves: 4

Ingredients

- 2 tablespoons avocado oil
- 1 large onion, minced
- 2 garlic cloves, minced
- 1 teaspoon ras el hanout spice blend or curry powder
- ¼ teaspoon cayenne pepper
- 1 teaspoon kosher salt
- 1 cup vegetable broth or water
- 1 tablespoon tomato paste
- 2 cups chopped eggplant
- 2 medium gold potatoes, peeled and chopped
- 4 ounces (113 g) tomatillos, husks removed, chopped
- 1 (14-ounce / 397-g) can diced tomatoes

Instruction:

1. Set the electric pressure cooker to the Sauté setting.
2. When the pot is hot, pour in the avocado oil.
3. Sauté the onion for 3 to 5 minutes, until it begins to soften.
4. Add the garlic, ras el hanout, cayenne, and salt.

5. Cook and stir for about 30 seconds.

6. Hit Cancel.

7. Stir in the broth and tomato paste.

8. Add the eggplant, potatoes, tomatillos, and tomatoes with their juices.

9. Close and lock the lid of the pressure cooker.

10. Set the valve to sealing.

11. Cook on high pressure for 3 minutes.

12. When the cooking is complete, hit Cancel and allow the pressure to release naturally.

13. Once the pin drops, unlock and remove the lid.

14. Stir well and spoon into serving bowls.

Nutrition facts: per, Serving (1½ cups) calories: 216 fat: 8g protein: 4g carbs: 28g sugars: 9g fiber: 8g sodium:

Crispy Dill Salmon

Prep Time: 05 min

Cook Time: 15 min

Serves: 4

Ingredients

- 1 cup panko bread crumbs
- 2 tablespoons olive oil
- 2 tablespoons snipped fresh dill
- 1/4 teaspoon salt
- 1/8 teaspoon pepper
- 4 Salmon fillets (6 ounces each)
- 1 tablespoon lemon juice Lemon wedges

Instruction:

1. Preheat the oven to 400 °.
2. Mix the first 5 ingredients.
3. Place the salmon in a 15 x 10 x 1-inch container.
4. Baking dish covered with cooking spray; Brush with lemon juice.
5. Top with breadcrumb mixture, pat to stick.
6. Bake uncovered on an upper rack of the oven until fish flakes easily with a fork, 12 to 15 minutes.
7. Serve with lemon wedges.

Nutrition facts: Calories 408 Total Fat 19.5g25% Saturated Fat 2.9g15%Cholesterol 78mg26% Sodium 427mg19% Total Carbohydrate 20.6g7% Dietary Fiber 1.5g5% Total Sugars 1.8g Protein 38.5g

Green Salad with Berries and Sweet Potatoes

Prep Time: 15 minutes

Cook Time: 20 minutes

Serves: 4

Ingredients:

For the vinaigrette:

- 1-pint blackberries
- 2 tbsp. red wine vinegar
- 1 tbsp. honey
- 3 tbsp. extra-virgin olive oil
- ¼ tsp. salt Freshly ground black pepper

For The Salad:

- 1 sweet potato, cubed
- 1 tsp. extra-virgin olive oil
- 8 cups salad greens (baby spinach, spicy greens, romaine)
- ½ red onion, sliced
- ¼ cup crumbled goat cheese

Instruction:

For The Vinaigrette:

1. In a blender jar, combine the blackberries, vinegar, honey, oil, salt, and pepper, and process until smooth.
2. Set aside.

For The Salad:

1. Preheat the oven to 425°F. Line a baking sheet with parchment paper.
2. Mix the sweet potato with the olive oil.
3. Transfer to the prepared baking sheet and roast for 20 minutes, stirring once halfway through, until tender.
4. Remove and cool for a few minutes.
5. In a large bowl, toss the greens with the red onion and cooled sweet potato, and drizzle with the vinaigrette.
6. Serve topped with 1 tbsp. goat cheese per serving.

Nutrition facts: Calories: 196 Carbohydrates: 21g Sugar: 10g

Blueberry and Chicken Salad

Prep Time: 10 minutes

Cook Time: 0 minute

Serves: 4

Ingredients:

- 2 cups chopped cooked chicken
- 1 cup fresh blueberries
- ¼ cup almonds
- 1 celery stalk
- ¼ cup red onion
- 1 tbsp. fresh basil
- 1 tbsp. fresh cilantro
- ½ cup plain, vegan mayonnaise
- ¼ tsp. salt
- ¼ tsp. freshly ground black pepper
- 8 cups salad greens

Instruction:

1. Toss chicken, blueberries, almonds, celery, onion, basil, and cilantro.
2. Blend yogurt, salt, and pepper.
3. Stir chicken salad to combine.
4. Situate 2 cups of salad greens on each of 4 plates and divide the chicken salad among the plates to serve.

Nutrition facts: Calories: 207 Carbohydrates: 11g Sugar: 6g

Buffalo Chicken Salads

Preparation Time: 7 minutes
Cooking Time: 3 hours
Servings: 5
Ingredients:

- 1½ pounds chicken breast halves
- ½ cup Wing Time® Buffalo chicken sauce
- 4 tsp. cider vinegar
- 1 tsp. Worcestershire sauce
- 1 tsp. paprika
- 1/3 cup light mayonnaise
- 2 tbsp. fat-free milk
- 2 tbsp. crumbled blue cheese
- 2 romaine hearts, chopped
- 1 cup whole-grain croutons
- ½ cup very thinly sliced red onion

Instruction:

1. Place chicken in a 2/4 slow cooker.
2. Mix together Worcestershire sauce, 2 tsp. of vinegar and Buffalo sauce in a small bowl; pour over chicken.
3. Dust with paprika.

4. Close and cook for 3 hours on a low-heat setting.
5. Mix the leftover 2 tsp. of vinegar with milk and light mayonnaise together in a small bowl at serving time; mix in blue cheese.
6. While chicken is still in the slow cooker, pull meat into bite-sized pieces using 2 forks.
7. Split the romaine among 6 dishes.
8. Spoon sauce and chicken over lettuce.
9. Pour with blue cheese dressing then add red onion slices and croutons on top.

Nutrition facts: Calories: 274 Carbohydrate: 11g Fiber: 2g

Orange Chicken Thighs

Prep time: 20 minutes

Cook time: 300 minutes

Serving: 4

Ingredients:

- Sliced fresh carrots,
- 2 cups Sliced tomatoes,
- 1 can Diced medium onion,
- 1 Tomato paste,
- 1 can Orange juice,
- 1-1/2 cup Chopped garlic cloves,
- 2 Dried basil,
- 2-3 teaspoons Sugar,
- 1-1/2 teaspoons Dried oregano,
- 1-1/2 teaspoon Dried thyme,
- 1-1/2 teaspoon Dried rosemary,
- 1-1/2 teaspoon Pepper,
- 1/2 teaspoon Grated orange zest,
- 2-3 teaspoons Debone chicken thighs,
- 8 Lemon juice,
- 2-3 tablespoons Baked bacon flakes, 4

Instructions :

1. Mix the first 12 items inside a 3-quart slow cooker.
2. Whisk in 1.5 teaspoon orange zest.
3. Now add the chicken on top and spoon the sauce over it.
4. Bake on low for 6-7 hours, or when the chicken is tender.
5. Transfer to a serving dish.
6. Add sauce over chicken thighs and whisk in 2-3 tablespoons lemon juice and leftover orange zest.
7. Scatter with bacon.
8. Then serve.

Nutrition Facts: 10g, Net Carbs: 15g, Protein: 25g, Sodium: 236mg

Artichoke Ratatouille Chicken

Prep time: 15 minutes

Cook time: 45 minutes

Serving: 4

Ingredients:

- Japanese eggplants,
- 3 Plum tomatoes,
- 4 Sweet yellow pepper,
- 1-2 Sweet red pepper,
- 1-2 Medium onion,
- 1 Quartered artichoke,
- 1 can Chopped thyme,
- 2-3 tablespoons Capers, drained,
- 2-3 tablespoons Olive oil,
- 2-3 tablespoons Chopped garlic cloves,
- 2 Creole seasoning,
- 1-2 teaspoons Debone chicken breasts,
- 1-1/2 pounds White wine,
- 1 cup Grated Asiago cheese,
- 1-1/4 cup Cooked pasta, optional

Instructions:

1. Preheat the oven to 350°Fahrenheit. 59

2. Cut the eggplants, plum tomatoes, peppers, and medium onion into 3/4-inch pieces; transfer them to a big bowl.
3. Mix in artichoke hearts, chopped thyme, capers, oil, chopped garlic cloves, and 1.5 teaspoon Creole seasoning.
4. Garnish the chicken with the rest of the Creole seasoning.
5. Now spoon veggies mixture over chicken inside a 13x9-inch baking dish sprayed with cooking oil.
6. Drizzle the wine over the vegetables.
7. Cook for 30 minutes, protected.
8. Uncover and cook for another 35-45 minutes, or until the chicken is lightly browned and the vegetables are tender.
9. Garnish with grated cheese.
10. Serve with cooked pasta if desired.

Nutritional Facts: Fat: 9g, Net Carbs: 15g, Protein: 28g, Sodium: 438mg

Vegan Chili with White Bean

Prep time: 10 minutes

Cook time: 45 minutes

Serving: 4

Ingredients:

- 2.5 tablespoons Canola oil,
- 1/4 cup Diced anaheim pepper,
- 2 cups Diced onion,
- 1 Chopped garlic cloves,
- 4 Quinoa, soaked,
- 1/2 cup Dried oregano,
- 4 teaspoons Ground cumin,
- 4 teaspoons Salt,
- 1 teaspoon Ground coriander,
- 1 teaspoon Ground pepper,
- 1 teaspoon Vegetable broth,
- 4 cups White beans,
- 15 ounces Chopped zucchini,
- 1 Diced cilantro,
- 1/4 cup Lime juice,

Instructions:

1. Heat oil inside a big pot on a medium flame.

2. Include the 1st 3 ingredients.

3. Cook, while constantly stirring, for 6 to 8 minutes, or until the veggies are tender.

4. Add quinoa, oregano, followed by cumin, salt, coriander, as well as pepper; cook them while stirring until fragrant, about 1 minute.

5. Whisk in the broth with beans.

6. Get the water to a boil.

7. Now reduce the flame and bring it to simmer.

8. Cook, moderately covered, for 20 minutes, while stirring occasionally.

9. Include zucchini; cover then cook, for 11 to 16 minutes or more, otherwise until the zucchini becomes tender and the chili has thickened.

10. Whisk in the cilantro with lime juice.

11. End up serving with lime wedges.

Nutrition Facts Fat: 11g, Net Carbs: 36g, Protein: 9g, Sodium: 529mg

Roasted Chickpea In Curry Bowl

Prep time: 15 minutes

Cook time: 45 minutes

Serving: 4

Ingredients:

- Olive oil, 2 tablespoons
- Curry powder, 1 tablespoon
- Salt, ½ teaspoon
- Head cauliflower, 1 medium
- Chickpeas, rinsed, 15 ounces
- Water, 1 ¼ cups
- Quinoa, rinsed, ⅔ cup
- Baby spinach, 4 cups
- Tahini, 2 tablespoons
- Lime juice, 1 teaspoon
- Clove Garlic, minced, 1
- Ground pepper, ⅛ teaspoon

Instructions:

1. Preheat the oven to 425°F.
2. Coat a large size baking sheet with the cooking spray.
3. In a medium-size mixing cup, combine the oil, some curry powder, and 1/2 teaspoon salt.

4. Toss in cauliflower and the chickpeas to coat.

5. Spread on prepared baking sheet.

6. Roast, stirring, for 20 mins, or till soft and brown.

7. Meanwhile, in a saucepan, add 1 1/4 cups of water, with quinoa and remaining 1/4 teaspoon salt.

8. Boil water over the medium-high flame.

9. Reduce heat to medium-low, cover, and cook for 12 to 15 mins, or till quinoa is tender.

10. Remove quinoa from heat and fluff with a fork.

11. Stir in the spinach, cover, and then allow to rest for 6 mins.

12. Meanwhile, in another bowl, combine tahini, 1 teaspoon lime zest, lime juice, 1 clove of garlic, pepper, and the remaining 2 tablespoons water.

13. Divide quinoa mixture into four dinner bowls.

14. Drizzle tahini dressing over cauliflower-chickpea mixture and serve to enjoy this recipe.

Nutritional Facts: Fat: 15g, Net Carbs: 43g, Protein: 13g, Sodium: 625mg

Pepper Steak Squash

Prep time: 10 minutes

Cook time: 30 minutes

Serving: 4

Ingredients:

- Beef broth, 1 can
- Soy sauce, 2.5 tablespoons
- Cornstarch, 3 tablespoons
- Canola oil, 2.5 tablespoons
- Beef flank steak, 1.5 pounds
- Green pepper, 1
- Sweet red pepper, about 1
- Zucchini, flaked, 2
- Onion, flaked, 1
- Garlic cloves, 3
- Snow peas, 1 cup
- Mushrooms, 1 cup
- Water chestnuts, 8.5 ounces
- Hot cooked rice, 1 bowl

Instructions:

1. Mix beef broth, soy sauce, including cornstarch inside a mixing bowl until smooth.
2. Place aside. Inside a big pan, warm 1 teaspoon oil over moderate flame.

3. Include beef and stir-fry for 3-4 minutes, or until the meat is properly cooked.

4. Take out from the skillet.

5. In the same pan, warm the remaining oil.

6. Include peppers and stir-fry for 2 minutes.

7. Include zucchini, onion with garlic; bake and stir for 2 minutes more.

8. Add snow peas and sliced mushrooms with water chestnuts.

9. Again, Stir-fry for 2 minutes, otherwise until crisp-tender.

10. Whisk cornstarch mixture, then add to skillet.

11. Now bring to a simmer while stirring until the sauce thickens, 1-2 minutes.

12. Transfer the meat to the pan; cook through.

13. End up serving with cooked rice.

Nutritional Facts Fat: 11g, Net Carbs: 16g, Protein: 18g, Sodium: 381mg

Flank Steak Beef

Prep Time: 10 minutes

Cook Time: 20 minutes

Serves: 4

Ingredients:

- 1 pound flank steaks, sliced
- ¼ cup xanthan gum
- 2 tsps. vegetable oil
- ½ tsp. ginger
- ½ cup soy sauce
- 1 tbsp. garlic, minced
- ½ cup water
- ¾ cup swerve, packed

Instructions:

1. Preheat the Air fryer to 390°F and grease an Air fryer basket.
2. Coat the steaks with xanthan gum on both sides and transfer them into the Air fryer basket.
3. Cook for about 10 minutes and dish out on a platter.
4. Meanwhile, cook the rest of the ingredients for the sauce in a saucepan.
5. Bring to a boil and pour over the steak slices to serve.

Nutrition facts: Calories: 372 Fat: 11.8 g Carbs: 1.8 g Sugar: 27.3 g Protein: 34 g

Sodium: 871 mg

French Onion Soup

Prep time: 10 minutes

Cook time: 30 minutes

Serves: 2

Ingredients:

- 6 onions, chopped finely
- 2 cups vegetable broth
- 2tbsp oil
- 2tbsp Gruyere

Instructions:

1. Place the oil in your Instant Pot and cook the onions on Saute until soft and brown.
2. Mix all the ingredients in your Instant Pot.
3. Cook on Stew for 35 minutes.
4. Release the pressure naturally.

Nutrition facts: Calories: 110;Carbs: 8 ;Sugar: 3 ;Fat: 10 ;Protein: 3 ;GL: 4

Dinner

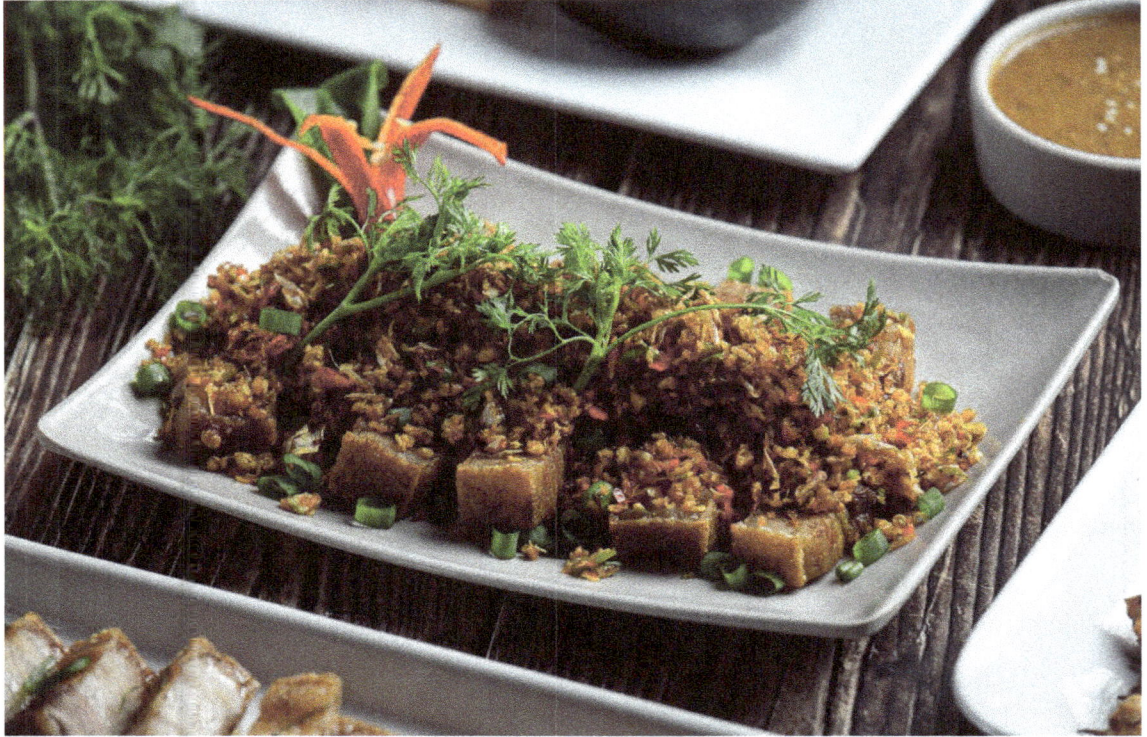

Baked Garlic Lemon Salmon

Prep Time: 5 minutes

Cook time: 15 minutes

Serves: 4

Ingredients:

- 3 tablespoons lemon juice
- 4 medium-sized salmon fillets
- ¼ cup unsalted butter, melted
- 2 cloves garlic, minced
- A handful of parsley, finely chopped
- Salt and pepper to taste

Instructions

1. Preheat the oven to 400°F (200°C).
2. Line a baking dish or tray with tin foil; grease with some cooking spray.
3. Place the salmon fillets over the baking dish.
4. Add the butter, garlic, lemon juice, salt and pepper to a mixing bowl.
5. Mix well.
6. Brush the salmon fillets with the butter sauce, reserving some sauce.
7. Bake for around 15 minutes, or until the salmon is easy to flake.
8. Bake for 2–3 minutes more if needed.
9. Brush with the reserved sauce and sprinkle some lemon juice on top.
10. Serve with chopped parsley on top.

Nutrition facts: Calories 350 Fat 25 g Total carbs 2 g Sugar 0.5 g, Protein 28.5 g Sodium 68 mg

Hearty Pumpkin Chicken Soup

Prep Time: 15 minutes

Cook Time: 35 minutes

Servings 6

Ingredients

- 1 small onion, thinly sliced
- 2 cloves garlic, minced
- 1 pound chicken breast, thinly sliced
- 1 tablespoon vegetable oil or coconut oil
- 1 medium zucchini, diced
- 1-inch piece ginger, peeled and minced
- ¾ pound pumpkin, cubed into ½-inch pieces
- 1 small chili or jalapeno pepper, seeded and thinly sliced
- 1 red bell pepper, seeded and thinly sliced
- 2 cups chicken broth
- 1 (14-ounce) can light coconut milk A handful of cilantro leaves Juice of 1 lime
- Salt and pepper to taste

Directions

1. Season the chicken slices with salt and pepper.
2. Heat the oil over medium-high heat in a large cooking pot.

3. Add the chicken and stir cook for 4–5 minutes to evenly brown.
4. Add the onion, ginger, and garlic and stir cook for 2–3 minutes until softened and translucent.
5. Add the zucchini and cubed pumpkin; stir well.
6. Add the chicken broth, coconut milk, bell pepper, chili or jalapeno pepper, and lime juice; stir again.
7. Bring to a boil, cover, and simmer over low heat for about 20 minutes, until the pumpkin is cooked well and softened.
8. Season with additional salt and pepper, if required.
9. Serve warm with cilantro leaves on top.
10. Note: You can store leftovers in an airtight container in the refrigerator for up to 3–4 days.
11. Simply re-heat in a cooking pot and serve.

Nutrition facts: Calories 231 Fat 13 g Total carbs 11.5 g Sugar 5 g, Protein 17 g Sodium 1207 mg

Colorful sweet potato salad

Prep Time: 5 minutes

Cook Time: 30 minutes

Servings: 4

Ingredients

- 450 g sweet potato
- Sea salt and black pepper, curry powder, to taste
- 1 ½ tbsp. olive oil
- 100 g baby spinach
- ½ organic lemon
- 30 g of walnuts
- ½ organic apple, green
- ½ teaspoon maple syrup
- 1 tbsp. vegetable stock
- 2 tbsp. quinoa, puffed, approx. 15 g
- ½ handful of chive flowers

Directions

1. Preheat the oven to 200 degrees (convection). Line a baking sheet with parchment paper.
2. Peel the sweet potato and cut into bite-sized pieces.
3. Mix with sea salt, black pepper, curry and 1 tbsp. oil and place on the baking tray, cook for about 20 minutes, turning occasionally, then leave to cool.
4. In the meantime, clean, wash and spin-dry the spinach. Halve the lemon, squeeze out the juice. Chop walnuts.

5. Wash the apple, cut into quarters and remove the core, cut into bite-sized pieces and drizzle with a little lemon juice.

6. For the dressing, stir together lemon juice, maple syrup, sea salt, pepper and oil vigorously.

7. Finally, put all the ingredients in a bowl and mix with the dressing. Then divide the salad on two plates, sprinkle the quinoa on top and garnish with the chives flowers.

8. Note: Quinoa (puffed) is already available in many supermarkets, but also in health food stores and health food stores.

Nutrition facts: Calories: 211 kcal Protein: 5.49 g Fat: 14.41 g Carbohydrates: 19.38 g

Barbecue Pork Loin

Prep Time: 10 minutes, plus 20 minutes marinating time

Cook Time: 35 minutes

Servings: 6

Ingredients

- 1½ pounds boneless pork sirloin roast
- 1 cup white vinegar
- 3 small garlic cloves, pressed
- 1 tbsp. creole seasoning
- ½ tsp smoked paprika
- ½ tsp cayenne pepper
- ½ cup chicken broth (here) or store-bought low-sodium chicken broth, plus more as needed
- ½ cup Barbecue Sauce, plus more for serving

Directions

1. Preheat the oven to 400°F.
2. In a medium bowl, combine the pork, vinegar, and garlic.
3. Set aside to marinate for 10 minutes.
4. Remove the pork from the marinade, shaking off any remaining vinegar, and transfer to a rimmed baking sheet.
5. Massage the pork all over with the Creole seasoning, paprika, and cayenne.
6. Cover and set aside for 20 minutes. In a Dutch oven, bring the broth to a simmer over high heat.

7. Add the pork and cook for 2 to 3 minutes per side, or until lightly browned. If the broth runs low, to keep the pork moist, add ¼ cup when turning.
8. Cover the pot, transfer to the oven, and cook for 30 minutes or until the pork is opaque.
9. Cover with the barbecue sauce, return to the oven, and cook for 5 to 7 minutes, or until a nice crust forms on the exterior.
10. Transfer the pork to a cutting board. Let rest for 5 to 10 minutes.
11. Slice the pork and serve with extra barbecue sauce.

Nutrition facts: Calories: 204 Total fat: 7 g Cholesterol: 75 mg Sodium: 134 mg

Ginger Halibut Bites

Prep time: 15 minutes

Cook time: 15 minutes

Serves: 4

Ingredients

- Lemon juice
- 4 teaspoons Halibut fillets
- 4 Minced gingerroot
- 1 teaspoon Salt
- 3/4 teaspoon Pepper
- 1/4 teaspoon Water
- 1/2 cup Brussels sprouts
- 10 ounces Red pepper flakes
- 1 tablespoon Canola oil
- 1 tablespoon Garlic cloves
- 5 Sesame oil
- 2 tablespoons Soy sauce
- 2 tablespoons

Instructions

1. Brush the halibut fillets with lemon juice.
2. Toss with some minced ginger, 1/4 teaspoon of salt, and freshly ground pepper.
3. Place the fish down from the skin side onto an oiled grill shelf.
4. Grill, covered, over medium heat for 6-8 mins, till the fish starts to flake effortlessly with a fork. Boil the water in a skillet over medium-high heat.
5. Stir in the Brussels sprouts with pepper flakes and any remaining salt if necessary.

6. Cook, covered, for 5-7 minutes, or until the vegetables are soft.

7. Meanwhile, heat oil into a skillet over a medium flame.

8. Cook until the garlic is golden brown. Using paper towels, drain it.

9. Drizzle halibut with sesame oil and some soy sauce.

10. Now serve with Brussels sprouts and fried garlic.

11. Serve with some lemon slices if needed.

Nutritional Facts Fat: 12g, Net Carbs: 7g, Protein: 24g, Sodium: 701mg

Sirloin Steak With Tomato & Pepper

Prep time: 15 minutes

Cook time: 35 minutes

Serves: 6

Ingredients

- Whole wheat flour 1/2 cup
- Salt,
- 3/4 teaspoon Pepper,
- Sirloin steak, chopped, 1-1/2 pounds
- Canola oil 3-4 tablespoons
- Chopped onion 1
- Chopped garlic clove.
- 1 Chopped tomatoes,
- 30 ounces Chopped green pepper,
- 2 Beef broth,
- 3-4 tablespoons Worcestershire sauce,
- 1.5 teaspoons Cooked rice, 1 bowl

Instructions

1. Combine the first 3 ingredients inside a large mixing bowl.
2. Add them with the beef, one at a time.
3. Mix gently to coat the beef with the mixture.
4. Warm the oil inside a Dutch oven at medium-high temperature.
5. Cook the beef in batches.
6. Include onion; bake and stir for 4-5 minutes, or until the onion is tender.
7. Now in a skillet, include garlic; cook for 1 minute.

8. Add tomatoes and again cook for few minutes.

9. Reduce the flame.

10. Now transfer the meat to skillet and Simmer, covered, for 11-16 minutes, or until the meat is tender.

11. Whisk in green peppers, beef broth, and sauce; cook covered for 11-15 minutes until the peppers are soft. Serve with rice.

Nutritional Facts Fat: 12g, Net Carbs: 17g, Protein: 27g, Sodium: 552mg

Italian Chicken

Prep time: 10 minutes

Cook time: 30 minutes

Serves: 4

Ingredients

- 5 chicken thighs
- 1 tbsp. olive oil
- 1/4 cup parmesan; grated
- 1/2 cup sun dried tomatoes
- 2 garlic cloves; minced
- 1 tbsp. thyme; chopped.
- 1/2 cup heavy cream
- 3/4 cup chicken stock
- 1 tsp. red pepper flakes; crushed
- 2 tbsp. basil; chopped
- Salt and black pepper to the taste

Instructions

1. Season chicken with salt and pepper, rub with half of the oil, place in your preheated air fryer at 350 °F and cook for 4 minutes.
2. Meanwhile; heat up a pan with the rest of the oil over medium high heat, add thyme garlic, pepper flakes, sun dried tomatoes, heavy cream, stock, parmesan, salt and pepper; stir, bring to a simmer, take off heat and transfer to a dish that fits your air fryer.

82

3. Add chicken thighs on top, introduce in your air fryer and cook at 320 °F, for 12 minutes.
4. Divide among plates and serve with basil sprinkled on top.

Nutritional Facts: Calories: 272; Fat: 9; Fiber: 12; Carbs: 37; Protein: 23

Parmesan-Topped Acorn Squash

Prep Time: 8 minutes

Cook Time: 20 minutes

Serves: 4

Ingredients

- 1 acorn squash (about 1 pound)
- 1 tablespoon extra-virgin olive oil
- 1 teaspoon dried sage leaves, crumbled
- ¼ teaspoon freshly grated nutmeg
- 1/8 teaspoon kosher salt
- 1/8 teaspoon freshly ground black pepper
- 2 tablespoons freshly grated Parmesan cheese

Instructions

1. Chop acorn squash in half lengthwise and remove the seeds. Cut each half in half for a total of 4 wedges. Snap off the stem if it's easy to do.
2. In a small bowl, combine the olive oil, sage, nutmeg, salt, and pepper. Brush the cut sides of the squash with the olive oil mixture.
3. Fill 1 cup of water into the electric pressure cooker and insert a wire rack or trivet.
4. Place the squash on the trivet in a single layer, skin-side down.
5. Set the lid of the pressure cooker on sealing.
6. Cook on high pressure for 20 minutes.
7. Once done, press Cancel and quick release the pressure.
8. Once the pin drops, open it.

9. Carefully remove the squash from the pot, sprinkle with the Parmesan, and serve.

Nutritional Facts: 85 Calories 12g Carbohydrates 2g Fiber

Fish & Chip Traybake

Prep time: 30/40 min

Cook time: 35 min

Serving: 4

Ingredients:

- 2 large sweet potatoes , cut into thin wedges
- 1 tbsp rapeseed oil
- 4 tbsp fat-free natural yogurt
- 2 tbsp low-fat mayonnaise
- 3 cornichons , finely chopped,
- 1 tbsp of the brine
- 1 shallot , finely chopped
- 1 tbsp finely chopped dill , plus extra to serve
- 300g frozen peas
- 50ml milk
- 1 tbsp finely chopped mint
- 4 cod or pollock loin fillets
- 1 lemon , cut into wedges, to serve

Instructions:

1. Heat the oven to 220C/200C fan/gas Toss the sweet potatoes with the oil and a little seasoning on a baking sheet and roast for 20 minutes.
2. Combine the yoghurt, mayonnaise, cornichons and reserved brine, shallots and dill with 1 tbsp cold water on the side.
3. Place the peas in a saucepan with the milk, bring to the boil and cook for 5 minutes.
4. Blend the mixture until coarsely pureed.

5. Stir in the mint and season to taste.

6. Set aside.

7. Add the cod or pollock to the pan with the sweet potatoes, season and bake for 10-15 minutes more or until cooked through.

8. Heat the pea mixture.

9. Sprinkle on some dill and serve the baking dish with the yogurt tartare and mushy peas.

Nutrition facts: 206 calories , 184 milligrams sodium, 6 grams trans fat, 20 grams protein, 4g fat

Pork In Chinese

Prep time: 10 min

Cook time: 7/8 min

Serves 2

Ingredients:

- pork lean meat 50 g
- frozen vegetables chinese mixture 100 g
- quality vegetable oil 15 g
- solamyl 5 g(potato powder)

Instruction

1. We clean the meat, cut it into strips, wrap it in solamyl.
2. Fry the meat in a hot pan.
3. Then add vegetables, a small amount of water and stew.
4. Lightly salt.

Nutrition facts: values Energy 295 kcal / Protein 10.2 g / P (phosphorus) 106 mg / K (potassium) 197.5 mg / Na (sodium) 40.2 mg

Coconut Chicken Curry

Prep Time: 10 Minutes

Cook Time: 40 Minutes

Serves: 6

Ingredients:

- 1 Small Sweet Onion
- 2 Tsps Minced Garlic
- 1 Tsp Grated Ginger
- 3 Tbsps Olive Oil
- 6 Boneless, Skinless Chicken Thighs
- 1 Tbsp Curry Powder
- ¾ Cup Of Water
- ¼ Cup Of Coconut Milk
- 2 Tbsps Cilantro, Chopped

Instructions:

1. Place A Medium Saucepan Or Skillet On Medium Heat, Add 2 Tablespoons Oil.
2. Add Chicken And Stir-Cook Until Evenly Brown, About 8-10 Minutes.
3. Set Aside.
4. Add Remaining Oil.
5. Add Onion, Ginger, Garlic, And Stir-Cook Until Softened, About 3-4 Minutes.
6. Mix In Curry Powder, Water And Coconut Milk.
7. Add Chicken, Stir The Mixture And Boil It.
8. Cover And Simmer The Mixture Over Low Heat For Another 25 Minutes Until Chicken Is Tender.

9. Serve Warm With Cilantro On Top.

Nutrition facts: Calories 258, Fat 13g, Phosphorus 151mg, Potassium 242mg, Sodium 86mg, Carbohydrates 2g, Protein 25g

Chicken and Veggie Soup

Prep Time: 15 Minutes

Cook Time: 25 Minutes

Serves: 8

Ingredients:

- 4 - cups cooked and chopped chicken
- 7 - cups reduced-sodium chicken broth
- 1 - pound froze white corn
- 1 - medium onion diced
- 4 - cloves garlic minced
- 2 - carrots peeled and diced
- 2 - celery stalks chopped
- 2 - teaspoons oregano
- 2 - teaspoon curry powder
- ½ - teaspoon black pepper

Instructions:

1. Include all fixings into the moderate cooker.
2. Cook on LOW for 8hours Serve over cooked white rice.

Nutrition facts: Calories: 220 Fat:7g Protein: 24g Carbs: 19g

Seafood And Andouille Medley

Prep Time: 5 Minutes

Cook Time: 40 Minutes

Serves: 3

Ingredients:

- 2 Andouille Sausages,

- Cut Crosswise Into ½ -Inch-Thick Slices

- ½ Stick Butter, Melted

- 2 Tomatoes, Pureed

- 2 Tbsps Fresh Cilantro, Chopped

- ½ Pound Skinned Sole, Cut Into Chunks

- 1/3 Cup Dry White Wine

- 1 Shallot, Chopped

- 2 Garlic Cloves, Finely Minced

- 1 Tbsp Oyster Sauce

- 3/4 Cup Clam Juice

- 20 Sea Scallops

Instructions:

1. Dissolve the butter in a heavy-bottomed pot over medium-high heat.

2. Heat the sausages until no longer pink, set aside.

3. Sauté the garlic and shallots in the same pan until they are softened; set aside.

4. Include the oyster sauce, pureed tomatoes, clam juice and wine; simmer for another 12 minutes.

5. Add the scallops, skinned sole and sausages.

6. Let it simmer, partially covered, for another 6 minutes.

7. Enjoy garnished with fresh cilantro. Bon appétit!

Nutrition facts: Calories 481, Protein 46.6g, Fat 26.9g, Carbs 5g, Sugar 1.1g

Chicken and Veggie Soup

Prep Time: 15 Minutes

Cook Time: 25 Minutes

Serves: 8

Ingredients:

- 4 - cups cooked and chopped chicken
- 7 - cups reduced-sodium chicken broth
- 1 - pound froze white corn
- 1 - medium onion diced
- 4 - cloves garlic minced
- 2 - carrots peeled and diced
- 2 - celery stalks chopped
- 2 - teaspoons oregano
- 2 - teaspoon curry powder
- ½ - teaspoon black pepper

Instructions:

3. Include all fixings into the moderate cooker.
4. Cook on LOW for 8hours Serve over cooked white rice.

Nutrition facts: Calories: 220 Fat:7g Protein: 24g Carbs: 19g

Ground Lamb with Peas

Prep Time: 15 Minutes

Cook Time: 55 Minutes

Serves: 4

Ingredients:

- One tablespoon coconut oil
- Three dried red chilies
- 1 (2-inch) cinnamon stick
- Three green cardamom pods
- ½ teaspoon cumin seeds
- One medium red onion, chopped
- 1 (¾-inch) piece fresh ginger, minced
- Four garlic cloves, minced
- 1½ teaspoons ground coriander
- ½ teaspoon garam masala
- ½ teaspoon ground cumin
- ½ teaspoon ground turmeric
- ¼ teaspoon ground nutmeg
- Two bay leaves
- 1-pound lean ground lamb
- ½ cup Roma tomatoes, chopped
- 1-1½ cups water

- 1 cup fresh green peas, shelled
- Two tablespoons plain Greek yogurt, whipped
- ¼ cup fresh cilantro, sliced
- Salt and freshly ground black pepper

Instructions:

1. In a Dutch oven, melt coconut oil on medium-high heat.
2. Add red chilies, cinnamon sticks, cardamom pods, and cumin seeds and sauté for around thirty seconds.
3. Add onion and sauté for about 3-4 minutes.
4. Add ginger, garlic cloves, and spices and sauté for around thirty seconds.
5. Add lamb and cook approximately 5 minutes.
6. Add tomatoes and cook approximately 10 min.
7. Stir in water and green peas and cook, covered approximately 25-thirty minutes.
8. Stir in yogurt, cilantro, salt, and black pepper and cook for around 4-5 minutes. Serve hot.

Nutrition facts: Calories: 430 Fat: 10g Carbohydrates: 22g Fiber: 6g Protein: 26g

Asian-Style Pan-Fried Chicken

Prep Time: 20 Minutes

Cook Time: 25 Minutes

Serves: 4

Ingredients:

- 12 ounces boneless, skinless chicken thighs, fat removed, cut into 2 or 3 pieces each
- One teaspoon low-sodium soy sauce
- One teaspoon dry rice wine
- 1-inch piece ginger, minced
- ½ cup cornstarch
- Three teaspoons canola oil, divided
- One lemon, cut into wedges

Instructions:

1. In a medium bowl, combine the chicken, soy sauce, rice wine, and ginger.
2. Toss and let sit for 15 minutes.
3. Toss the chicken again, and drain the liquid from the bowl.
4. One at a time, put the chicken pieces in the cornstarch to coat.
5. In a medium skillet over medium-high heat, heat 1½ teaspoons of oil, add half of the chicken to the pan, and cook until golden brown on one side, about 3 to 5 minutes.
6. Flip and continue to cook on the opposite side until the chicken is cooked through and is golden brown.
7. Transfer the chicken to a plate wrinkled with paper towels to cool.

8. Add the remaining 1½ teaspoons of oil, and repeat the cooking process with the remaining chicken thighs.

9. Serve garnished with lemon wedges.

Nutrition facts: Calories: 198 Total Fat: 7g Cholesterol: 71mg Carbohydrates: 16g Fiber: 0g Protein: 17g Phosphorus: 148mg Potassium: 218mg Sodium: 119mg

Dessert

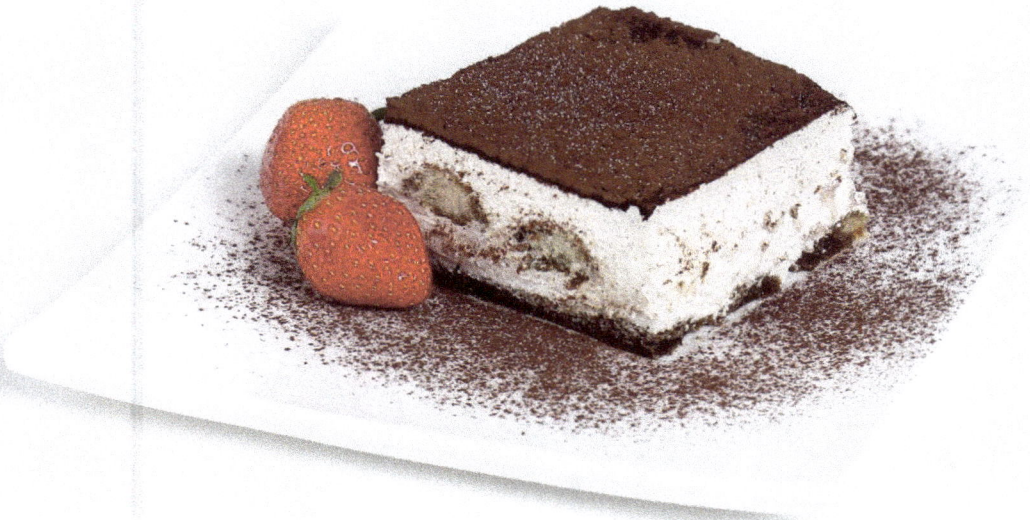

Jalapeno and Cheddar Muffins

Prep Time: 9 Minutes

Cook Time: 35 Minutes

Servings: 8

Ingredients:

- cups finely diced raw cauliflower
    - 2 tablespoons minced jalapeno
    - 2 eggs, beaten
    - 2 tablespoons melted butter
    - 1/3 cup grated parmesan cheese
    - 1 cup grated mozzarella cheese
    - 1 cup grated cheddar cheese
    - 1 tablespoon dried onion flakes
    - ¼ teaspoon salt
    - ¼ teaspoon black pepper
    - ½ teaspoon garlic powder
    - ½ teaspoon baking powder
    - ¼ cup coconut flour

Instructions:

1. Preheat the oven to 375°F.
2. Combine the cauliflower, jalapeno, eggs, add melted butter in a medium bowl.
3. Add the grated cheeses and mix well.

4. Stir in the onion flakes, salt, pepper, garlic powder, baking powder, and coconut flour until thoroughly combined.

5. Divide the batter evenly between 12 greased muffin cups.

6. Bake for 30 minutes or until golden brown.

7. Turn off the oven and leave the muffins inside for about an hour.

8. Remove from the oven.

9. Cool on a wire rack.

10. Serve and enjoy!

Nutrition facts: Calories: 130 Total Carbs: 13g Fat: 6g Protein: 19g 74.   Low Carb

Honey Raisin Cookies

Prep Time: 11 Minutes

Cook Time: 29 Minutes

Servings: 6

Ingredients:
- 1/2 cup butter, softened
- 1/2 cup honey
- 1 egg
- 1 teaspoon vanilla
- 1 cup whole wheat flour
- 1 teaspoon baking powder
- 1/4 teaspoon salt
- 1/2 cup oats
- 1/2 cup raisins
- 1/2 cup chopped walnuts

Instructions:
1. Combine the first four ingredients and mix well.
2. Combine the next four ingredients and add to the honey-butter mixture.
3. Add the raisins and chopped walnuts.
4. Bake at 350°F for 12-15 minutes or until just lightly golden brown.

Nutrition facts: Calories: 227 Fat: 12g Carbohydrates: 28g Protein: 4g

Sweet Potato Bread

Preparation time: 15 minutes

Cooking time: 45 minutes

Servings 4

Ingredients:

- 1 large peeled and diced sweet potato
- 1 Tbsp of ground flaxseeds
- 3 Tbsp of water
- 2 and ½ cups of almond flour
- 1 Teaspoon of dried thyme
- 1 Teaspoon of fresh chopped rosemary
- ½ Teaspoon of sea salt
- 2 Tbsp of extra-virgin olive oil

Instructions:

1. Preheat your oven to around 350 F.
2. Steam your sweet potatoes into a steamer basket in an instant pot or boil steam it in a steamer basket above the stove on top of boiling water for around 6 to 9 minutes.
3. Mix the flax seeds with water in a deep bowl and set it aside for around 10 minutes.
4. Mix again very well and mash the cooked potatoes with a potato masher or with a fork.
5. Add the rest of the ingredients and then add the rest of the ingredients and mix all the ingredients together very well.
6. Form the dough from your mixture and transfer your dough to a lined parchment and roll the dough with a rolling pin into around ½ inch of thickness.
7. Bake the dough for about 40 to 45 minutes.

8. Once the bread becomes brown, remove it from the oven and set it aside to cool down for around 20 minutes.

9. Cut the bread into rectangles.

10. Serve and enjoy!

Nutrition facts: Calories: 100 | Fat: 3 g | Carbohydrates: 11g | Fiber: 1 g | Protein: 4.9 g

Raspberry And Cashew Balls

Preparation time: 15 minutes

Cooking time: 0 minutes

Servings 14

Ingredients:

- 1⅓ Cup of raw cashews or almonds
- ¼ Cup of cashew or almond butter
- 2 Tablespoons of coconut oil
- 2 Pitted Medjool dates, pre-soaked into hot water for about 10 minutes
- ½ Teaspoon of vanilla extract
- ¼ Teaspoon of kosher salt
- ½ Cup of freeze-dried and lightly crashed raspberries
- 1 Cup of chopped dark chocolate

Instructions:

1.   In a high-powered blender or a Vitamix; combine the cashews or almonds with the butter, the coconut oil, the Medjool dates, the vanilla extract and the salt and pulse on a high speed for about 1 to 2 minutes or until the batter starts sticking together.
2. Pulse in the dried raspberries and the dark chocolate until your get a thick mixture.
3. With a tablespoon or a small cookie scoop, divide the mixture into balls of equal size.
4. Arrange the balls in a container or a zip-top bag in a refrigerator for about 2 weeks or just serve and enjoy your delicious cashew balls!

Nutrition facts; Calories: 108.2| Fat: 7.4 g | Carbohydrates: 5.9g | Fiber: 1.3g |Protein: 3 g

Apple and Cinnamon Muffins

Preparation time: 15 minutes

Cooking time: 20-25 minutes

Servings: 12 muffins

Ingredients:
- 2 cups almond flour
- 1 teaspoon baking powder
- 1/2 teaspoon baking soda
- 1 teaspoon ground cinnamon
- 1/4 teaspoon nutmeg
- 1/4 teaspoon salt
- 1/4 cup melted coconut oil
- 1/4 cup sugar-free sweetener
- 2 eggs
- 1 teaspoon vanilla extract
- 1 cup grated apples

Instructions:
1. Preheat the oven to 350°F and prepare a muffin tin with liners.
2. In a large bowl, mix almond flour, baking powder, baking soda, cinnamon, nutmeg, and salt.
3. In another bowl, whisk together melted coconut oil, sugar-free sweetener, eggs, and vanilla extract.
4. Gradually add the wet ingredients to the flour mixture and stir until well combined.

5. Add grated apples and mix well.
6. Divide the batter evenly among the muffin liners.
7. Bake for 20-25 minutes or until golden and cooked through.
8. Allow the muffins to cool before serving.

Nutritional values per muffin: Calories: 140 Carbohydrates: 7g Fat: 12g Protein: 5g

Chocolate Avocado Pudding

Preparation time: 10 minutes

Cooking time: 0 minutes (in the refrigerator)

Servings: 2

Ingredients:
- 1 ripe avocado
- 1/4 cup unsweetened cocoa powder
- 1/4 cup unsweetened almond milk
- 2 teaspoons sugar-free sweetener (or to taste)
- 1/2 teaspoon vanilla extract
- Pinch of salt

Instructions:
1. Cut the avocado in half, remove the pit, and scoop out the flesh.
2. Place the avocado flesh, cocoa powder, almond milk, sugar-free sweetener, vanilla extract, and salt in a blender.
3. Blend until smooth and creamy.
4. Transfer the pudding to two bowls or glasses.
5. Cover with plastic wrap and refrigerate for at least 1-2 hours.
6. Serve chilled.

Nutritional values per serving: Calories: 190 Carbohydrates: 12g Fat: 15g Protein: 4g

Sugar-Free Lemon Ricotta Cake

Preparation time: 15 minutes

Cooking time: 40-45 minutes

Servings: 8

Ingredients:

- 2 cups low-fat ricotta cheese
- 4 eggs
- Grated zest of 2 lemons
- Juice of 1 lemon
- 1/2 cup sugar-free sweetener
- 1 teaspoon vanilla extract
- 1/4 cup almond flour

Instructions:

1. Preheat the oven to 350°F and grease a cake pan or line it with parchment paper.
2. In a bowl, whisk together the ricotta cheese, eggs, lemon zest, lemon juice, sugar-free sweetener, vanilla extract, and almond flour.
3. Pour the mixture into the prepared cake pan.
4. Bake in the oven for 40-45 minutes or until the cake is golden and cooked through.
5. Allow the cake to cool completely before serving.

Nutritional values per serving: Calories: 130 Carbohydrates: 4g Fat: 9g Protein: 10g

Sugar-Free Vanilla Ice Cream

Preparation time: 5 minutes

Cooking time: 0 minutes (in the freezer)

Servings: 4

Ingredients:
- 2 cups heavy cream
- 1 cup unsweetened almond milk
- 2 teaspoons sugar-free sweetener
- 2 teaspoons vanilla extract

Instructions:
1. In a bowl, mix together the heavy cream, almond milk, sugar-free sweetener, and vanilla extract.
2. Pour the mixture into an ice cream maker and follow the manufacturer's instructions to make the ice cream.
3. If you don't have an ice cream maker, pour the mixture into a freezer-safe container and stir well every 30 minutes until creamy.
4. Transfer the sugar-free vanilla ice cream to a sealed container and freeze for at least 2-3 hours or until firm.
5. Serve the ice cream with desired toppings.

Nutritional values per serving: Calories: 180 Carbohydrates: 2g Fat: 18g Protein: 2g

Sugar-Free Oatmeal Raisin Cookies

- Preparation time: 10 minutes
- Cooking time: 12-15 minutes
- Servings: approximately 16 cookies

Ingredients:

- 1 cup oats
- 1/4 cup almond flour
- 1/2 teaspoon baking powder
- 1/2 teaspoon ground cinnamon
- 1/4 teaspoon salt
- 1/4 cup melted coconut oil
- 1/4 cup sugar-free sweetener
- 1 egg
- 1 teaspoon vanilla extract
- 1/4 cup raisins

Nutritional values per cookie:

- Calories: 75
- Carbohydrates: 6g
- Fat: 5g
- Protein: 2g

Instructions:

1. Preheat the oven to 350°F and line a baking sheet with parchment paper or lightly grease it.
2. In a bowl, mix together oats, almond flour, baking powder, cinnamon, and salt.
3. In another bowl, whisk together melted coconut oil, sugar-free sweetener, egg, and vanilla extract.
4. Add the wet ingredients to the dry ingredients and mix until well combined.
5. Add raisins and mix well.
6. Take small portions of the dough and form round cookies.

7. Place the cookies on the prepared baking sheet.

8. Bake for 12-15 minutes or until the cookies are golden around the edges.

9. Allow the cookies to cool completely before serving.

Conclusion

In conclusion, the book "Diabetic Diet Cookbook" written by Gena Miller represents a comprehensive and informative resource for those looking to adopt a diabetes-friendly diet and improve their overall health. Through a wide range of delicious and nutritious recipes, the author provides a practical and accessible approach to managing daily nutrition, demonstrating that a diabetes diet doesn't have to be tasteless or monotonous. The book begins by providing a solid foundation of knowledge on diabetes, including the basic principles of the glycemic index, the importance of blood glucose control, and specific nutritional guidelines for diabetic patients. This introductory section is valuable for those seeking a better understanding of their condition and the implications that diet can have on diabetes management.

What truly sets the book apart and makes it exceptional is its extensive collection of balanced and flavorful recipes. Gena Miller offers readers a variety of options for breakfast, lunch, dinner, and snacks, ranging from classics to innovative culinary creations. Each recipe is carefully designed to include nutrient-rich ingredients and ensure proper balance of carbohydrates, proteins, and fats. Furthermore, detailed nutritional information is provided to assist readers in monitoring calorie intake and meal composition.

Another notable aspect of the book is its emphasis on accessibility and practicality of the recipes. Gena Miller takes into account the time constraints and demands of modern life, providing tips for meal prepping and pantry organization. This makes it easier to follow the proposed diet, allowing readers to seamlessly incorporate healthy habits into their daily routine.

Lastly, the "Diabetic Diet Cookbook" by Gena Miller stands out for its clarity and ability to communicate complex information in a simple and understandable manner. Detailed instructions and helpful illustrations make meal preparation easy, even for those with limited culinary experience.

In summary, "Diabetic Diet Cookbook" is an essential work for anyone looking to follow a healthy and balanced diet for diabetes, offering tasty recipes and practical advice to help readers improve blood glucose control and promote long-term healthy living.

www.ingramcontent.com/pod-product-compliance
Lightning Source LLC
Chambersburg PA
CBHW081200020426
42333CB00020B/2571